CSID ELIMINATION DIET COOKBOOK FOR BEGINNERS

Symptom Relief for Congenital Sucrase-Isomaltase Deficiency and Improved Gastrointestinal Health with Healthy Low-Sucrose, Low-Starch Recipes

Eddy Beckett M.D.

The content in this book is provided solely for general information purposes. While we make every effort to keep the information up to date and correct, we make no express or implied representations or warranties about the completeness, accuracy, reliability, suitability, or availability of the publication or the information, products, services, or related graphics contained in the publication for any purpose. Your reliance on such material is thus entirely at your own risk.

We shall not be liable for any loss or harm, including without limitation, indirect or consequential loss or damage, or any loss or damage deriving from loss of data or profits originating from or in connection with the use of this publication.

This publication may contain links to websites that are not under our control. We have no influence on the nature, content, or accessibility of other websites. The presence of any links does not constitute a suggestion or endorsement of the ideas expressed within them.

Every effort is taken to maintain the publication operational. Nevertheless, we accept no responsibility for, and will not be accountable for, the publication being momentarily unavailable owing to technical reasons beyond our control.

Table of Contents

INTRODUCTION

An uncommon genetic condition known as Congenital Sucrase-Isomaltase Deficiency (CSID) affects the small intestine and the digestive system as a whole. Enzymes sucrase and isomaltase are essential for the digestion of certain sugars; in this disorder, one or both of these enzymes is lacking. Isomaltase aids in the digestion of certain complex carbs, whereas sucrose, which is present in table sugar, is broken down by sucrase.

Malabsorption and other gastrointestinal problems manifest in people with CSID because their digestive systems are unable to break down these sugars correctly. The severity of the illness might differ among affected individuals, and it is present from birth. When it comes to controlling their digestive health, some people may have moderate symptoms while others may have much more severe problems.

Malnutrition, gas, bloating, diarrhea, and stomach discomfort are all possible symptoms of CSID. The level of enzyme insufficiency and the kinds and quantities of carbohydrates eaten can determine the severity and start of symptoms. The autosomal recessive inheritance pattern of CSID indicates that a kid can only be afflicted if both parents possess a faulty gene.

Combining clinical assessment with laboratory testing and molecular genetic testing to identify specific gene mutations linked with the disorder is the standard procedure for diagnosing CSID. In order to reduce the consumption of problematic sugars and promote optimum nutrient absorption, dietary adjustments are generally the focus of management efforts once a diagnosis is made. In certain instances, enzyme replacement treatment could also be explored.

Maintaining good nutrition and managing symptoms while living with CSID may necessitate strong collaboration between healthcare providers, especially dietitians, and patients. Despite the lack of a cure, researchers are making strides in understanding the disorder's genetic foundation, which bodes well for future diagnostic improvements and treatment approaches. Improving the quality of life for people with Congenital Sucrase-Isomaltase Deficiency requires a holistic and tailored approach to treatment.

CHAPTER 1: WHAT IS CONGENITAL SUCRASE-ISOMALTASE DEFICIENCY?

An extremely rare genetic disorder known as congenital sucrose isomerase deficiency (CSID) disrupts normal digestion, particularly in the small intestine. It seems that sucrase and isomaltase, two essential enzymes, aren't part of the digestive team. In digestion, these enzymes are the unsung heroes responsible for breaking down carbohydrates. While isomaltase aids in the digestion of some complex carbohydrates, sucrose—the sugar found in table sugar—is handled by sucrase.

Dealing with CSID is like having a digestion crew that is understaffed from the very beginning. They have a plethora of unpleasant symptoms, including gastrointestinal issues, since they are unable to digest these carbohydrates correctly. Imagine if you will: gas, diarrhea, stomach ache, bloating, and so forth. Malnutrition is a serious issue when their systems aren't absorbing nutrients properly. This condition is inherited in an autosomal recessive fashion, meaning it is somewhat inherited from one generation to the next. In other words, a child can only have CSID if both parents inherit a defective gene.

Diagnostic procedures for CSID include standard medical exams, laboratory testing, and, in certain cases, genetic testing to identify the offending gene(s). Managing a CSID diagnosis typically requires a planned approach to eating. To do this, one must discover strategies to reduce the intake of troublesome sugars while simultaneously increasing the intake of nutrients. To speed things along, enzyme replacement treatment may be necessary at times.

In order to keep things under control, people living with CSID must make sensible decisions while eating and work together with healthcare professionals, particularly dietitians. There may not be a silver bullet for CSID just yet, but scientists are studying the virus's genetic makeup in the hopes of developing more accurate diagnostic tools and, ultimately, effective therapies. At the moment, our focus is on finding our way around food while keeping CSID in mind, and we're working on creating a tailored plan to help those living with this rare genetic condition.

Importance of Dietary Management

Conditions like Congenital Sucrase-Isomaltase Deficiency (CSID) make dietary control a crucial part of people's life. What those afflicted eat has a direct impact on their day-to-day functioning and emotional state. Paying close attention to food choices becomes essential for symptom relief and good nutritional absorption when dealing with CSID, as it hinders the digestion of certain carbohydrates.

Reducing sugar consumption is a key component of nutritional management for people with isomaltase and sucrase insufficiency, as these sugars are difficult for the body to digest. This often entails cutting back or eliminating sweets that cause issues, such sucrose and specific types of complex carbs. By following these steps, people can lessen the chances of suffering from CSID symptoms as gas, diarrhea, and stomach discomfort.

The development of an effective and long-lasting eating regimen requires close cooperation between patients and healthcare providers, notably registered dietitians. Professionals in this field may advise people on how to make healthy food choices, where to find sweets that can be harmful, and how to meet all of their nutritional requirements. The prevention of malnutrition, which occurs when the body fails to absorb vital nutrients, and the promotion of general health both depend on this collaboration.

To help digest sugars, some people with CSID may look into enzyme replacement treatment in addition to changing their diet. Nevertheless, the daily food choices are the bedrock of efficient management. The key is to eat a varied and healthy diet while also being aware of the particular restrictions caused by the illness.

Dietary treatment is important for people with CSID for reasons beyond only alleviating symptoms; it also improves their quality of life. People may live better, more satisfying lives if they take charge of their nutrition, prevent food-related pain, and make educated eating choices. Dietary management is becoming more complex as a result of genetic condition research and understanding, which highlights the importance of individualized and thorough treatment for people with CSID and similar illnesses.

Development of CSID

The sugar-digesting enzymes sucrase and isomaltase in the hereditary condition known as Congenital Sucrase-Isomaltase Deficiency (CSID), are either absent or severely impaired. The susrase-isomaltase (SI) gene mutation is a key genetic component in the development of cystic fibrosis. The sucrase and isomaltase enzymes are encoded by this gene; mutations in this gene can lead to enzymes that do not operate properly or have reduced functionality.

Because CSID is passed down through generations in an autosomal recessive fashion, it takes a defective gene from both sets of parents for a person to develop the disease. People who carry the gene mutation from parent to child often do not exhibit any symptoms themselves but are able to pass the gene on to their offspring. With each pregnancy, the chances of a kid inheriting two mutant genes and developing CSID increase by 25% when both parents are carriers.

When people start eating a wide variety of foods that are high in sugar, the symptoms of CSID usually start to show themselves in early infancy. Abdominal discomfort, bloating, gas, and diarrhea are some of the gastrointestinal symptoms that can arise from a lack of sucrase and isomaltase, which causes the malabsorption of certain sugars.

It is common practice to combine clinical assessment with laboratory testing and genetic testing when diagnosing CSID. By delving into the condition's genetic origins, medical experts can identify the particular SI gene mutations that validate the diagnosis.

There is currently no known cure for cystic fibrosis, however the disease can be managed with dietary changes, enzyme replacement treatment, and behavioral alterations. Dietitians and gastroenterologists are key members of the healthcare team that individuals with CSID collaborate with to develop individualized plans to reduce symptoms and maximize nutrient intake.

Research is being conducted to gain a better knowledge of the genetic variants linked to CSID. This might result in better diagnosis tools and more precise treatment strategies. Because CSID is inherited, genetic counseling can help affected people and their families understand the illness better and make more educated decisions about family planning.

CHAPTER 2: ENZYME DEFICIENCY

Enzyme deficit is the fundamental problem with Congenital Sucrase-Isomaltase deficit (CSID). In particular, the enzymes sucrase and isomaltase are either absent or insufficient in those who have CSID. The small intestine relies on these enzymes to absorb carbohydrates, among their many important functions in digestion. In contrast to isomaltase, which facilitates the digestion of certain complex carbs, sucrose is broken down into glucose and fructose by sucrase.

Inadequate levels of these vital enzymes set off a chain reaction of gastrointestinal problems. Malabsorption occurs when the body does not have enough of the enzymes sucrase and isomaltase to break down sugars properly. Abdominal discomfort, gas, bloating, and diarrhea are some of the gastrointestinal symptoms that can result from malabsorption. In short, the body's capacity to absorb vital nutrients from food is impaired due to the enzyme deficit, which interferes with regular digestive function.

Due to its hereditary nature, CSID causes enzyme deficiencies, the severity of which might vary from person to person. The autosomal recessive inheritance pattern requires the presence of a faulty gene in both parents for the condition to manifest in a child. The digestive experience of a person with an enzyme shortage begins at birth and continues throughout their growth.

In order to manage CSID, it is common to take measures to rectify the enzyme deficit. Individuals may be prescribed enzyme supplements as part of enzyme replacement treatment to make up for the deficiency in their body's natural sucrase and isomaltase. In order to alleviate symptoms and improve overall digestive function, this treatment intervention seeks to restore the balance of enzymes necessary for optimal sugar digestion.

Essential components of CSID management include comprehending and resolving the complexities of enzyme insufficiency. Healthcare providers can better assist their patients in achieving optimal health by collaborating with them to develop individualized treatment plans that improve symptom management and the digestive system's ability to handle sugars efficiently.

Hereditary Nature of CSID

Congenital Sucrase-Isomaltase Deficiency (CSID) is a genetic disorder that runs in families due to its hereditary nature. Because CSID is an autosomal recessive disorder, it takes two copies of the faulty gene from each parent for a kid to have the condition. Carrier individuals usually do not show signs of CSID themselves, but they do have one normal gene and one mutant gene.

There is a 25% probability that a kid born to a parent who is a carrier will also acquire the CSID gene mutation. Because of this genetic interaction, CSID tends to cluster in families; those who have the disease typically have at least one parent who is either a carrier or has the disease themselves.

Affected people and their families must understand the genetic component of CSID.

Because it tells you how likely it is that you will pass the faulty gene on to your children and grandchildren, genetic counseling is a valuable resource. Family planning decisions and the safety of other family members can be better understood with the help of this therapy.

Although CSID's genetic basis provides insight into its heritability, the degree to which symptoms manifest can differ even among carriers of the same mutation. This provides more evidence that CSID's expression and effect may be impacted by other environmental or genetic variables, further complicating its hereditary dynamics.

Our understanding of CSID is being further advanced by research into the precise genetic alterations linked to the disorder. There is hope for earlier diagnosis and more precise treatments as genetic testing advances. Therefore, the familial context of CSID is informed by its hereditary origin, which also serves as a focus point for current attempts to enhance diagnostic and treatment methods by unraveling the genetic complexity of the disorder.

Symptoms and Impact on Digestion

A variety of symptoms affecting the digestive process are experienced by those living with Congenital Sucrase-Isomaltase Deficiency (CSID). This hereditary disorder revolves around the inability or insufficiency of the digestive enzymes sucrase and isomaltase, which are in charge of sugar breakdown. Consequently, those suffering from CSID frequently encounter a multitude of gastrointestinal symptoms, which can vary from minor discomfort to more severe problems.

Patients suffering with CSID frequently report abdominal discomfort, gas, and bloating. These unpleasant feelings are caused by a chain reaction of digestive problems that begin when the body tries to digest sweets incorrectly. Another common concern is diarrhea, which occurs when the carbohydrates that are not digested cause the intestines to absorb too much water, leading to loose and watery stools.

Beyond these short-term effects, CSID can hinder digestion and, by extension, nutritional absorption. Malnutrition might develop over time as a result of the body's inability to absorb vital nutrients due to impaired sugar breakdown. Fatigue, weakness, and other health issues may be one result of this nutritional deficit, which can have far-reaching effects on general health.

People living with CSID need to be mindful of their food choices on a daily basis because of the effects on digestion. When trying to control symptoms, some sweets become off-limits or need careful portion control. Consequently, meal preparation becomes an involved and methodical procedure, frequently including healthcare providers and nutritionists to guarantee a healthy and well-rounded diet with little discomfort.

The main objective of controlling CSID is to achieve a balance, even if the symptoms and effects on digestion might differ in intensity across individuals. Symptom relief through dietary changes, meeting nutritional requirements, and, when required, investigating treatment therapies are all part of this equilibrium. Individuals can improve their digestive health and quality of life by tackling the difficulties of CSID holistically.

CHAPTER 3: CSID-FRIENDLY FOODS

The daily lives of those managing Congenital Sucrase-Isomaltase Deficiency (CSID) revolve around making the proper dietary choices. Foods that are less likely to cause CSID symptoms include those that are low in sugar, an ingredient that the body has trouble breaking down because of enzyme deficiencies in sucrase and isomaltase. Because they might cause unpleasant gastrointestinal symptoms, meals rich in sucrose and other complex carbs should be limited or avoided.

Because they contain fewer of the troublesome sugars, starchy foods such as rice, potatoes, and maize are usually well-tolerated by people with CSID. Also, CSID-friendly foods include strawberries, bananas, and blueberries because they don't have as many sugars, which might make your digestive system upset.

People with CSID usually consume protein-rich meals like chicken, fish, and lean meats because they give all the nutrients they need without all the sugar. Because CSID and lactose intolerance may not often occur together, those who need to limit their lactose consumption may find that almond or coconut milk are viable replacements.

Dietitians and other healthcare providers can help patients choose CSID-friendly meals that will meet their nutritional needs while reducing their symptoms. It's not enough to simply cut out specific meals; you also need to come up with novel substitutions and well-rounded eating regimens to improve your health in general.

Specialty goods made with troublesome sugars in mind may be an option for some people with CSID. Commercially accessible items that address dietary limitations related to CSID and sweeteners that are compatible with the disease are examples of what this category encompasses. The aim is to establish a long-term, pleasurable eating regimen that caters to the specific requirements of people with CSID, encouraging a healthy connection with food and the successful management of symptoms.

Dietary Recommendations

A crucial part of dietary treatment for people with Congenital Sucrase-Isomaltase Deficiency (CSID) is avoiding meals that are heavy in sugars that the body has trouble digesting, since this can worsen symptoms. Foods containing sucrose, which is present in table sugar, are among the leading candidates. A variety of sugary foods and drinks, as well as sweets, can irritate the gastrointestinal tract and cause diarrhea in people with CSID.

Additionally, those with CSID should exercise caution while consuming complex carbs like those in wheat, barley, and rye. Abdominal discomfort and bloating may result from consuming these grains because of the carbohydrates they contain, which may be difficult to digest. It may be necessary to restrict or replace foods that include these grains with alternatives that are more accepted. These foods include bread, spaghetti, and baked goods.

For those with CSID, dairy products can add additional layer of difficulty, particularly if they are lactose intolerant. It may be necessary to limit high-lactose dairy products like milk and ice cream and look into lactose-free alternatives in order to keep calcium intake steady without triggering gastrointestinal problems.

Making educated decisions based on knowledge of the sugar content of various meals is essential for CSID dietary management. In order to develop a tailored strategy for identifying and managing trigger foods, it is essential to collaborate with healthcare specialists, such as dietitians. Creating a balanced and pleasurable diet that responds to the particular requirements of persons with CSID is the objective, not an exhaustive list of items to avoid or limit. The goal is to promote digestive comfort and general well-being.

Balancing Meals in Managing CSID

A balanced and healthy diet, in addition to avoiding items that cause Congenital Sucrase-Isomaltase Deficiency (CSID), is essential for the successful management of this condition. As people with CSID strive to reduce symptoms while making sure they get all the nutrients they need, maintaining a balanced diet becomes an important part of the overall strategy.

Incorporating sources of easily digested carbs is essential for maintaining meal balance for those with CSID. Due to their reduced sugar content, foods such as rice, potatoes, and cooked vegetables are often well-tolerated. As a steady supply of energy that won't worsen symptoms, they can be the basis of a meal.

Another way to improve meal balance is to eat carbs with foods that are high in protein. You can get all the amino acids you need from lean meats, poultry, and fish without adding a ton of sugar to your diet. Protein aids in maintaining general health and also stabilizes blood sugar levels, which means you'll have more energy to get you through the day.

Healthy fats are a concentrated source of energy that may enhance the flavor and fill you up. Nutritious fats, such as olive oil, almonds, seeds, and avocados, are an important part of a healthy diet. In addition to assisting in food absorption, fats can make you feel full, which can help you regulate your portion sizes.

To make sure you receive a variety of vitamins, minerals, and fiber, it's best to focus on vegetables, particularly ones with less sugar. In addition to being essential for general wellness, these components have the potential to enhance gastrointestinal health and digestion. Natural sweetness may be added without overloading the digestive system by using fruits with reduced sugar content or by choosing small servings.

The development of a diet plan that satisfies dietary requirements within the constraints placed by CSID requires close cooperation between the patient and healthcare providers, especially registered dietitians. For optimal health, digestive ease, and a balanced approach to meals, it's important to watch portion sizes, eat smaller portions more frequently, and drink enough of water.

Portion Control and Timing

Controlling portion sizes and eating at regular intervals are two important steps in the complex dance of controlling Congenital Sucrase-Isomaltase Deficiency (CSID). In order to manage symptoms, it is crucial for patients with CSID to carefully watch the portion sizes. In order to ease the body's digestive system, it is generally advised to eat smaller meals more often throughout the day. Spreading out food consumption across many smaller meals might help individuals limit their intake of harmful sugars, which in turn reduces the chances of experiencing unpleasant symptoms like diarrhea and stomach discomfort.

For individuals navigating CSID, the timing of meals is equally important. The digestive process and symptoms might be better managed with the support of a regular eating routine. Eating at regular intervals gives your digestive system a routine, which in turn makes it easier for your body to absorb lower sugar loads. Blood sugar levels and the secretion of digestive enzymes can both be helped by eating more steadily.

Mastering portion management goes beyond just cutting back on unhealthy food intake. It entails picking foods that are rich in nutrients and promote health without putting too much strain on the digestive system. It is crucial to work with healthcare providers, especially dietitians, to customize serving sizes and meal schedules to each person's unique requirements and way of life.

It is also critical to be cognizant of one's own tolerance levels and to modify serving quantities according to one's own reactions. By tailoring their treatment to their specific needs, people with CSID are able to eat well while reducing their risk of gastrointestinal distress. To effectively incorporate portion control and mindful meal scheduling into the daily routine, it is important to maintain open contact with healthcare experts, check progress often, and be flexible when it comes to making dietary modifications.

CHAPTER 4: MANAGEMENT OF CSID

The complexities of one's own digestive environment is crucial for those navigating the complex world of self-management with Congenital Sucrase-Isomaltase Deficiency (CSID). Dietary knowledge is fundamental to individual management, since people traverse a terrain where certain carbohydrates might pose a threat. An essential map on this path is working closely with healthcare providers, especially nutritionists. Collaboratively, they develop an individual plan to reduce symptom triggers and meet nutritional requirements.

A key component in maintaining this equilibrium is controlling portion sizes; eating smaller meals more often becomes a tactic. Spreading out the digestive activity throughout the day helps people avoid the bloating and gas that might come from eating a big, sugary meal all at once. A complicated dance of combining nutrient richness with digestive comfort, it's not just about limitation but about developing a palette of meals that nourish without overpowering.

As a possible ally in the management of individual CSIDs, enzyme replacement therapy enters the scene. Some people find that these supplements work in tandem with their bodies' digestive enzymes to help break down carbohydrates that are too complex for their bodies to handle on their own. The fact that results could differ highlights the importance of tailoring treatment to each person's unique genetic makeup and way of life.

Lifestyle factors are an integral part of CSID management, going beyond only the food. Essential elements include cultivating a mindful eating habit, engaging in regular physical exercise, and learning to handle stress. When eaten at regular intervals, meals become choreographed to the body's natural digestion pattern. An often-overlooked but vital element in maintaining the digestive system's fluid equilibrium is hydration.

However, there is more to individual CSID management than just the tactics. It covers the emotional terrain of dealing with an illness that involves daily cycles, food choices, and genetics. A lifeline of understanding and encouragement may be found in support networks, whether they take the form of family, friends, or other CSID fighters in online groups.

An individual's mental health, lifestyle choices, and food choices all come together in perfect harmony as they take center stage as conductors in this intricate self-management symphony. The path from a challenge to an ever-changing investigation of health and resilience is being shaped by the growing understanding of CSID and the role that individuals play in navigating this complex issue.

Expert Opinion for CSID Patients

Medical experts in the field of Congenital Sucrase-Isomaltase Deficiency (CSID) work together as a team to give patients individualized recommendations based on their specific condition. Expertise of dietitians, who are vital in developing unique eating regimens, is a key component of this process. Their expertise aids people in navigating the food maze, determining which foods promote healthy eating and which ones bring on symptoms. Adjustments can be made in response to individual reactions and changing requirements through regular discussions with dietitians.

If you are planning a family or are interested in learning more about the genetics of CSID, a genetic counselor may be a great asset in your professional guidance arsenal. In order to help people make educated decisions about family planning, these specialists give detailed information on the chances of passing on the mutant gene.

By working together with patients, gastroenterologists who focus on gastrointestinal problems do comprehensive evaluations and investigate possible treatment options. They may help people understand enzyme replacement therapy by explaining its ins and outs, answering queries, and shedding light on its possible advantages.

Mental health specialists, such as psychologists, may be a great resource when it comes to managing one's lifestyle. Mental health can suffer when living with a chronic illness like CSID; these experts can help with stress management, coping mechanisms, and building resilience.

Experts recommend that people with CSID have regular checkups and talk to their healthcare providers about any concerns they may have. An active strategy for managing this hereditary problem includes keeping an eye on symptoms, checking nutritional status, and dealing with any new issues as they arise.

In the end, the combined expertise and experience of these healthcare experts equips persons with CSID to deal with the challenges of their illness by providing them with information, encouragement, and a thorough strategy for overall health. The collaboration between these experts shows their shared goal of improving CSID patients' quality of life by helping them cope with their symptoms and develop a positive attitude about their health.

Exercise and CSID

Exercise has an important and multi-faceted role in the complex world of Congenital Sucrase-Isomaltase Deficiency (CSID) management, which contributes to overall health. Although physical activity does not cure CSID's enzymatic weaknesses, it helps the digestive system and makes you feel better overall.

To keep your digestive system in good working order, it's a good idea to exercise often. As food travels through the digestive system, the regular muscular contractions that occur during exercise may help keep things moving along smoothly. Exercise can be a proactive measure for those with CSID who may struggle with gastrointestinal symptoms to promote digestive function.

People dealing with long-term health issues, such as CSID, greatly benefit from exercising not just for their physical health, but also for their mental and emotional well. In cases when digestive issues are already present, the stress-relieving benefits of exercise may be especially welcome. Walking, running, yoga, or any kind of exercise may help with both the physical and mental aspects of resilience, so it's a win-win.

Nevertheless, every person with CSID has unique demands and limits, thus exercise regimens should be tailored to their specific condition. It is important to engage with healthcare specialists, such as gastroenterologists or fitness experts, to create an exercise plan that is specific to each person's health state and goals, as not everyone can safely participate in intense or high-impact activities.

In order to keep their digestive systems healthy, people with CSID must stay hydrated throughout activity. Some people with CSID may already be concerned about symptoms like constipation, and dehydration can make them worse.

Exercise does not cure CSID's enzyme deficits, but it improves digestive function, lowers stress, and boosts general health, thus it can be an important part of a comprehensive strategy for dealing with this hereditary disorder. People with CSID may take charge of their health and wellness by creating personalized fitness programs and working together with healthcare providers to achieve their goals.

Hydration and CSID

Individuals may support their digestive health by the simple yet effective avenue of staying hydrated, which is crucial in the holistic care of Congenital Sucrase-Isomaltase Deficiency (CSID). In order to promote proper digestive function, it is crucial for individuals with CSID to be adequately hydrated, as the breakdown of certain carbohydrates might be difficult for them. For some people living with this genetic disorder, constipation is already a problem, and dehydration can make it worse.

As it helps maintain a healthy fluid balance in the digestive tract, water gradually becomes an invaluable ally for people with CSID. Stools are easier to pass through the digestive system when they are well hydrated, which may alleviate the pain of constipation. Because fluid loss can occur as a result of CSID symptoms, such as diarrhea, it is very important to hydrate in order to prevent dehydration.

Hydration affects general health in addition to the digestive system. A practical and approachable part of self-care for people with CSID is making sure they drink plenty of fluids, especially because they may have to deal with a complicated interaction between food restrictions and possible gastrointestinal pain. In addition to promoting digestive health, it aids in preventing dehydration and its symptoms, including lethargy and low energy.

People with CSID can tailor their approach to staying hydrated by thinking about things like weather, how active they are, and what they like. Although water is the most common way to stay hydrated, other drinks such as herbal teas or infused water can also help with fluid consumption. Individualized hydration techniques help people with CSID find a happy medium between promoting digestive health and making fluid consumption a habit that they can stick to.

People with CSID can tailor their hydration plan to their unique health needs and dietary limitations with the help of their healthcare providers. As part of a comprehensive strategy for controlling CSID and supporting overall health, regular monitoring and open communication with healthcare experts help make hydration an essential tool.

CHAPTER 5: COPING WITH DIGESTIVE DISCOMFORT

Individuals controlling Congenital Sucrase-Isomaltase Deficiency (CSID) must constantly deal with intestinal discomfort. Because of the difficulties caused by the lack of the sucrase and isomaltase enzymes, pain management techniques are an integral part of everyday living. Understanding personal triggers and creating coping strategies that are specific to each person's needs is an important part of helping those with CSID.

When dealing with gastrointestinal pain, dietary changes are crucial. People whose systems have trouble digesting sugars can reduce their consumption of these foods by being mindful of portion sizes and meal choices. This usually entails cutting down or drastically reducing your intake of particular complex carbs and meals that are heavy in sugar.

Dietitians and other healthcare providers play a crucial role in working with patients to develop individualized eating programs that address both nutritional requirements and symptoms management. Some people with CSID may also want to look into enzyme replacement treatment, in addition to changing their diet. This entails supplementing the diet with enzymes to help digest carbohydrates more efficiently and make up for the deficit. The efficacy of enzyme replacement therapy in reducing pain varies from patient to patient, although it is generally a useful technique. Lifestyle factors are also a part of developing coping mechanisms. Improve your digestion by sticking to a regular meal schedule, eating mindfully, and drinking enough of water. Because stress can worsen symptoms in people with CSID, practicing stress management strategies like yoga or meditation may further assist in reducing the effects of stress on the digestive system. For both the mental and physical challenges that come with living with CSID, having a support system of loved ones or friends nearby may be invaluable. When others dealing with similar issues get together to share stories, advice, and words of encouragement, it may build a sense of community and strength. Dealing with gastrointestinal distress in CSID is, in the end, an ever-changing and growing experience. The quality of life for those dealing with this hereditary illness can be improved by a holistic strategy that includes regular communication with healthcare experts, continual self-awareness, and a willingness to adapt to individual requirements.

Adaptable Lifestyle Tips

Managing symptoms and maintaining general well-being can be greatly assisted by adopting specific lifestyle suggestions while negotiating the intricacies of Congenital Sucrase-Isomaltase Deficiency (CSID). Setting up a regular and personalized eating regimen is an important part. People with CSID can take better care of their digestive health if they work closely with healthcare providers, particularly dietitians, to develop a tailored eating plan that meets their specific needs.

One important way that people with CSID can improve their quality of life is by practicing mindful eating. Improving digestion and lowering the risk of pain can be achieved by being mindful of hunger signals, eating deliberately, and appreciating every meal. Incorporating moderate exercise into your daily routine on a regular basis can also help your digestive system and your health in general.

Another important aspect of CSID management is staying hydrated. A more regular fluid balance in the digestive tract may alleviate constipation and other related symptoms, therefore it's important to drink enough of water. Making informed decisions about hydration alternatives that work with dietary limitations is crucial. Seeking guidance from healthcare practitioners can help folks make the right choices.

People with CSID must prioritize stress management practices since stress worsens gastrointestinal symptoms. The digestive system can benefit from a more relaxed condition, which can be achieved by practices like yoga, deep breathing, or meditation.

Managing CSID effectively requires constant attention to detail, one of which is the development of a support network. If you or someone you know is going through a tough time, finding a support group or community online may be a great place to talk things out, get advice, and feel less alone.

The most important thing for people with CSID to do for their health is to stay in touch with their healthcare professionals. An active and cooperative approach to controlling this hereditary illness may be achieved by keeping them updated on symptom patterns, making necessary adjustments to food plans, and communicating any worries or difficulties that may occur. All things considered, people with CSID are able to live full lives despite their condition when they include these lifestyle guidelines into their daily routines.

CHAPTER V: HEALTHY LOW-SUCROSE, LOW-STARCH RECIPES CSID RECIPES

BREAKFAST RECIPES FOR CSID

Tortilla Scrambled Egg and Cheese

Ingredients

1 large egg

1 teaspoon milk

1 1/2 teaspoons butter

1 (7 inch) flour tortilla

2 slices jalapeno pepper jack cheese

How to Make

Whisk egg and milk together in a small bowl.

Melt butter in a skillet over medium heat. Pour in egg mixture and tilt skillet until egg covers the skillet. Cook until egg is set, about 2 minutes. Place flour tortilla over egg, and carefully flip egg and tortilla so that the tortilla is now on the bottom.

Place cheese slices over egg. Cook until tortilla is crisp, 3 to 4 minutes. Cover skillet and cook until cheese is melted, 1 to 2 minutes.

Fried Egg Tortilla

Ingredients

2 teaspoons butter

1 large egg

1/4 teaspoon taco seasoning, or to taste

1 1/2 ounces shredded Cheddar cheese, divided

1 (6 to 7-inch) flour tortilla

How to Make

In a 10-inch nonstick skillet, melt butter over medium heat, and swirl the pan to coat the bottom evenly.

Carefully break egg into buttered skillet and cook until egg white is opaque and egg is firm enough to turn, about 1 minute.

Turn egg over, being careful not to break yolk; sprinkle with taco seasoning and about half of cheese.

Gently place tortilla over egg and cheese, and cook about 1 minute. Using a silicone egg turner, flip the egg and tortilla, as one.

Sprinkle remaining cheese on top of the egg, and continue cooking until the egg is done to your liking and the tortilla is warm and toasty, about 2 minutes.

Slide tortilla and egg to a serving plate and serve warm

Easter Breakfast Casserole

Ingredients

cooking spray

1 pound bacon

8 large eggs

2 cups milk

3 cups shredded Cheddar cheese

¼ cup diced onion

¼ cup diced green bell pepper

1 (16 ounce) package frozen hash brown potatoes, thawed

How to Make

Preheat the oven to 350 degrees F (175 degrees C). Lightly grease a 7x11-inch casserole dish.

Fry bacon in a large, deep skillet over medium-high heat until evenly browned, about 10 minutes. Drain on a paper towel-lined plate. Crumble.

Beat together eggs and milk in a large bowl. Mix in cheese, bacon, onion, and green pepper. Stir in thawed hash browns. Pour mixture into prepared casserole.

Cover with aluminum foil and bake in preheated oven for 45 minutes. Uncover and bake until eggs have set, another 30 minutes.

Cauliflower Rice Pilaf

Ingredients

2 tablespoons unsalted butter

2/3 cup diced shallots

2/3 cup chopped fresh white mushrooms

3 tablespoons shredded carrots

1/2 teaspoon turmeric

1/8 teaspoon curry powder

1/8 teaspoon paprika

2 cloves garlic, minced

1/2 cup white wine

2 teaspoons chicken flavor bouillon base, such as Better Than Bouillon® Roasted Chicken Base

1 pound frozen riced cauliflower

salt and freshly ground black pepper, to taste

1/4 cup minced fresh parsley, plus more for garnish

How to Make

Melt butter in a skillet over medium heat. When butter sizzles, add diced shallots and cook about 2 minutes. Add chopped mushrooms and cook, stirring occasionally, about 3 minutes.

Add carrots, and sprinkle on turmeric, curry powder, and paprika. Stir in minced garlic and cook until fragrant, about 30 seconds.

Add white wine and chicken flavor bouillon base. Stir until chicken base is dissolved into the liquid. Cook, stirring occasionally, about 3 minutes. See Cook's Note.

Add frozen riced cauliflower, and use a fork to break up any clumps. Cook, stirring occasionally, until all the liquid is evaporated and cauliflower is tender, 5 to 8 minutes.

Season with salt and pepper, to taste. Stir in fresh minced parsley and place in a serving dish. Garnish with additional parsley, if desired.

Leftover Corn Chowder

Ingredients

1 tablespoon butter

1 large yellow onion, diced

1 teaspoon kosher salt

2 slices bacon, chopped

1/2 red bell pepper, seeded and diced

2 stalks celery, diced

2 cloves garlic, minced

2 chipotle peppers in adobo sauce, minced

1 (16 ounce) bag frozen corn

4 cups chicken stock

3/4 cup heavy whipping cream

1 1/2 cups leftover cooked chicken or other protein

1 tablespoon chopped cilantro or other garnish

How to Make

Heat butter in a soup pot over low heat until melted. Increase heat to medium-low, add onion and salt, and cook and stir until onion is translucent, about 5 minutes.

Stir in bacon, red pepper, celery, and garlic; cook and stir until bacon is crisp, about 5 minutes.

Add chipotle peppers, corn, and chicken stock to soup pot; increase heat to medium and simmer for 20 minutes.

Stir in cream and chicken. Cook until hot, about 5 minutes. Serve in bowls and garnish with cilantro.

Tuna and Artichoke Wraps

Ingredients

2 (5-ounce) cans tuna, drained

1 (7 1/2-ounce) jar artichoke hearts, drained and chopped

1 mini cucumber, chopped

1/2 cup chopped grape tomatoes

1/3 cup mayonnaise

1/2 teaspoon ground mustard

1 teaspoon garlic salt

1 lemon, zested

2 tablespoons fresh lemon juice

3 (10-inch) sun-dried tomato basil tortillas

6 lettuce leaves

6 tablespoons French-fried onions

How to Make

Stir tuna, artichokes, cucumber, tomatoes, mayonnaise, mustard, garlic salt, lemon zest, and lemon juice together in a bowl.

Lay out tortillas on a work surface; lay 2 lettuce leaves on each tortilla. Spoon tuna mixture in a line across the middle of each tortilla; top tuna with 2 tablespoons French-fried onions. Fold opposing edges of tortilla to overlap the filling. Roll 1 of the opposing edges around the filling creating a burrito.

Chilaquiles with Homemade Tomato Sauce

Ingredients

16 (6-inch) corn tortillas

2 cups oil, or as needed for frying

1 teaspoon kosher salt, plus more to taste

2 cups water

2 guajillo chiles, stems and seeds removed

1 white onion, quartered

3 cloves garlic

4 ripe tomatoes, quartered

2 jalapenos, halved

1 teaspoon ground cumin

1 (14.5 ounce) can fire-roasted diced tomatoes

2 teaspoons red wine vinegar

1 tablespoon olive oil

4 large eggs

1/2 cup crumbled queso fresco

1 avocado, sliced

1/4 cup crema

sliced radish, hot sauce, chopped cilantro, for garnish (optional)

How to Make

Cut each tortilla into 8 wedges. Heat oil to 350 degrees F (180 degrees C) in a large pot over medium-high heat. Add tortillas to fry in batches, taking care not to crowd the pot. Cook, stirring constantly until golden and crispy, 1 to 2 minutes. Remove from oil with a slotted spoon and drain well on paper towels. Sprinkle with salt to taste immediately. Repeat with remaining tortillas.

In a large saucepan, add water and guajillo chiles. Bring mixture to a boil over high heat, reduce temperature, and simmer until chiles soften, about 5 minutes. Return heat to medium-high and add onion, garlic, tomatoes, jalapenos, cumin, and 1 teaspoon salt. Cook, stirring occasionally, until onion has softened, about 10 minutes.

Remove from heat and carefully pour mixture into a blender or food processor. Add canned tomatoes, vinegar, and olive oil. Remove center from the lid to allow steam to escape and blend until smooth, about 1 minute, scraping down the sides as necessary.

In a large skillet over medium heat, add 1 cup of sauce and bring to a simmer, stirring often. Add 1/4 of the chips and cook about 3 minutes, stirring frequently, until the chips are well-coated in sauce and fully heated through. Place chips on a plate.

In a separate small skillet, heat 1/2 tablespoon butter over medium heat. Crack an egg into the butter and cook over easy or as desired. Add egg to chips and top with queso fresco, avocado, crema, and any other desired toppings.

Easy Cabbage and Bean Soup

Ingredients

2 tablespoons olive oil, plus more for drizzling

2 leeks, white and light green parts only, chopped

3/4 cup sliced carrots

3 cloves garlic, minced

1 1/2 quarts low-sodium vegetable broth

1/4 cup tomato paste

2 teaspoons dried Italian herb seasoning

salt and freshly ground black pepper to taste

1 pound cabbage, chopped

1 pinch red pepper flakes (optional)

2 (15 ounce) cans great Northern beans

fresh thyme sprigs for garnish (optional)

How to Make

Heat olive oil in a Dutch oven over medium heat. Add leeks and carrots, and cook, stirring frequently, about 3 minutes. Stir in garlic and cook until fragrant, about 30 seconds.

Pour in vegetable broth, stir in tomato paste and Italian seasoning, and bring to a boil. Reduce heat to low, cover, and simmer until vegetables are tender, about 10 minutes.

Using an immersion blender, puree the vegetables and liquid. Season with salt and pepper.

Increase heat to medium and bring to a boil. Stir in cabbage, red pepper flakes, and a couple more pinches of salt, if desired. Bring to a boil, reduce heat, and simmer until cabbage is tender, 20 to 25 minutes.

Stir in beans and simmer until beans are heated through, about 5 minutes more.

Serve warm, garnished with fresh thyme sprigs, if desired, and drizzled with olive oil.

Roasted Garlic Pasta

Ingredients

2 tablespoons finely chopped Italian parsley

1 lemon, zested

1 tablespoon lemon juice, or more to taste

1/2 teaspoon crushed red pepper flakes

1/4 cup peeled garlic cloves

1/2 cup extra-virgin olive oil

salt and freshly ground black pepper to taste

6 ounces angel hair pasta

3 ounces pecorino Romano cheese, grated, plus more for serving

How to Make

Preheat the oven to 375 degrees F (190 degrees C). Add garlic to a small oven-safe dish; pour olive oil on top to submerge the garlic. Cover the dish with a lid or foil.

Bake garlic in the preheated oven for 1 hour.

Add parsley, lemon zest, lemon juice, and red pepper flakes to a large bowl.

At the 50-minute mark, bring a large pot of salted water to a boil; add pasta and cook until tender with a bite, 4 to 5 minutes. Drain; set aside to keep warm.

Remove roasted garlic from the oven, and carefully pour off the oil into the bowl with parsley mixture. Add in roasted garlic, leaving cloves intact, or crushing some or all of them. Stir in cheese. Season to taste with salt and black pepper.

Stir pasta into the bowl with sauce, coating each and every noodle. Divide between 2 bowls. Sprinkle with a little more cheese if desired, and enjoy.

Hungarian Layered Cabbage

Ingredients

1 large head Savoy cabbage

1 tablespoon vegetable oil

1 red onion, diced

1 large clove garlic, minced, or more to taste

salt and freshly ground black pepper to taste

1 pound ground pork

1 tablespoon sweet paprika

1/3 cup water

1 teaspoon vegetable oil

3/4 cup uncooked white rice

1 1/2 cups water

2 cups sour cream

How to Make

Separate cabbage leaves, rinse, and remove the hard ribs by cutting closely along the center ribs on both sides of each leaf with a sharp knife; discard ribs. Bring a large pot of salted water to a boil. Add cabbage leaves, and cook until tender, 15 to 20 minutes; drain.

Preheat the oven to 350 degrees F (180 degrees C). Grease an 8x11-inch baking dish.

Meanwhile, heat 1 tablespoon vegetable oil in a skillet over low heat. Add onions, garlic, and a pinch of salt. Cook, stirring, until onions are soft and translucent, about 3 minutes.

Add pork and season with paprika, salt, and pepper. Cook, stirring frequently, about 5 minutes.

Pour in water, cover, and simmer until most of the water has evaporated, 15 to 20 minutes.

Meanwhile, heat 1 teaspoon vegetable oil in a saucepan over medium heat; add rice and toast until the grains are shiny, stirring frequently, about 1 minute. Pour in 1 1/2 cups water and a little salt. Bring to a boil, cover pot, and turn heat down to low. Cook until rice is tender and water is absorbed, 15 to 20 minutes. Turn off heat.

Line the prepared baking dish with 1/2 of the cabbage. Spread 1/2 of the cooked rice over the cabbage, followed by a layer of 1/2 of the cooked meat. Add another layer of 1/2 of the remaining cabbage, followed by a layer of remaining rice and meat; cover with remaining cabbage. Spread sour cream evenly over the top.

Bake in the preheated oven until casserole is heated through and sour cream is starting to lightly brown, 30 to 35 minutes

Sauteed Cabbage and Peppers

Ingredients

3 tablespoons olive oil

½ head red cabbage, chopped

½ onion, chopped

1 small red bell pepper, chopped

1 small yellow bell pepper, chopped

salt and ground black pepper to taste

How to Make

Heat olive oil in a large skillet over high heat; cook and stir cabbage, onion, red bell pepper, and yellow bell pepper in the hot oil, stirring every 30 seconds, until tender, 5 to 7 minutes. Season with salt and pepper.

Tomato Toast with Sriracha Mayo

Ingredients

1 tablespoon mayonnaise

3/4 teaspoon lime juice

1/2 teaspoon Sriracha sauce

2 slices bread

1 large heirloom tomato, chopped or sliced

2 teaspoons everything bagel seasoning, or to taste

How to Make

In a small bowl, mix together mayonnaise, lime juice, and sriracha sauce. Set aside.

Toast bread in a toaster or toaster oven. Top with tomato, sprinkle with everything bagel seasoning to taste, then drizzle with sriracha mayo.

LUNCH RECIPES FOR CSID

Grilled Flounder

Ingredients

1/4 cup olive oil

2 cloves garlic, minced

2 teaspoons lemon zest

2 tablespoons fresh lemon juice

2 teaspoons smoked paprika

1/4 teaspoon celery salt

4 (2 ounce) flounder filets

How to Make

Whisk olive oil, garlic, lemon zest, lemon juice, smoked paprika, and celery salt together in a bowl. Pour into a resealable plastic bag.

Add flounder filets, coat with the marinade, squeeze out excess air, and seal the bag. Marinate in the refrigerator for 30 minutes.

Preheat an outdoor grill for medium-high heat and lightly oil the grate.

Cook the flounder on the preheated grill until the filets flake easily with a fork, about 4 minutes per side.

Tuna-Stuffed Pita Pockets

Ingredients

2 teaspoons freshly-squeezed lime juice

1 teaspoon Dijon mustard

1/2 teaspoon white sugar

2 tablespoons olive oil

1 (5-ounce) can solid white Albacore tuna in water, drained and chunked

1 1/2 tablespoons chopped red onion

1 tablespoon peeled, seeded, and chopped cucumber

1 tablespoon chopped fresh parsley

1 tablespoon drained capers (optional)

salt and freshly ground black pepper to taste

1 (6-inch) whole wheat pita bread

2 lettuce leaves

6 cherry tomatoes, halved

2 tablespoons sliced Kalamata olives

2 tablespoons crumbled feta cheese

How to Make

Stir lime juice, Dijon, and sugar together in a small bowl. Gradually whisk in olive oil until dressing thickens slightly.

Place tuna in a separate bowl; add onion, cucumber, parsley, and capers. Drizzle dressing over tuna mixture and stir gently, trying to keep tuna chunky. Season with salt and pepper.

Slice pita in half and open halves to form pockets. Place leaf lettuce in the pita halves, and spoon in tuna mixture. Top with tomatoes, olives, and feta cheese. Serve immediately.

Cornmeal-Crusted Cod

Ingredients

12 cod filets

1/4 cup lime juice

2/3 cup cornmeal

2/3 cup all-purpose flour

salt and freshly ground black pepper to taste

1/2 cup olive oil

1/4 cup butter

How to Make

Rinse cod filets with water. Pat fish dry.

Place lime juice in a shallow bowl. Whisk cornmeal, flour, salt, and pepper together in a separate shallow bowl.

Heat oil and butter in a large cast-iron skillet over medium heat. Using tongs, dip cod into lime juice; allow excess to drip off. Press fish into cornmeal mixture to coat on all sides; set aside on a plate.

Fry cod in the hot skillet until crispy golden brown, 2 to 3 minutes. Turn and fry until fish flakes easily with a fork and is golden brown on the other side; about 1 minute more. Cooking time will depend on thickness of filets. You may have to fry in batches.

Remove fish to a wire rack set over a drip tray to catch any excess oil. Serve immediately.

Grilled Rockfish Sandwich

Ingredients

1/4 cup light beer

1/4 cup Dijon mustard

1 teaspoon garlic powder

1 teaspoon lemon pepper seasoning

4 (6 ounce) rockfish filets

4 hamburger buns

4 romaine lettuce leaves

4 tomato slices

4 tablespoons mayonnaise

How to Make

Whisk beer, Dijon mustard, garlic powder, and lemon pepper seasoning together in a bowl. Pour into a resealable plastic bag.

Add rockfish filets, coat with the marinade, squeeze out excess air, and seal the bag. Marinate in the refrigerator for 30 minutes.

Preheat an outdoor grill for medium-high heat and lightly oil the grate.

Grill rockfish on the preheated grill until filets flake easily with a fork, about 4 minutes per side. Toast hamburger buns on the grill until grill marks for, about 2 minutes.

Divide mayonnaise between toasted hamburger buns. Top each bun with one portion of cooked rockfish, one tomato slice, and one lettuce leaf.

Seasoned Pan-Fried Cod

Ingredients

1 teaspoon smoked paprika

1/2 teaspoon kosher salt

1/4 teaspoon garlic powder

1/4 teaspoon onion powder

1/8 teaspoon celery seed

2 (6 ounce) cod filets, patted dry

1 tablespoon unsalted butter

1 tablespoon lemon juice

2 teaspoons chopped parsley (optional)

How to Make

Add smoked paprika, salt, garlic powder, onion powder, and celery seed to a bowl; stir until evenly combined. Season cod filets on all sides with mixture and place on a plate.

Melt butter in a skillet over medium-high heat. Add cod and fry for 3 minutes.

Turn filets over, add lemon juice, and fry until cod flakes easily with a fork, about 2 minutes more. Transfer to a serving plate; garnish with parsley.

Salmon Stir-Fry

Ingredients

1 pound salmon filet

salt and freshly ground black pepper to taste

2 tablespoons sesame oil

1 red bell pepper, cut into bite-sized pieces

1 yellow bell pepper, cut into bite-sized pieces

1 onion, cut into bite-sized pieces

1 cup fresh broccoli florets

1 tablespoon chopped fresh garlic

1 tablespoon ginger paste

2 tablespoons hoisin sauce

1/2 cup shredded carrots

How to Make

Heat a cast iron skillet over medium-high heat. Season salmon with a sprinkle of salt and pepper.

Cook salmon until fish flakes easily with a fork, 3 to 5 minutes on each side. Remove from skillet and set aside.

Heat sesame oil in a wok or heavy skillet over high heat. Add red pepper, yellow pepper, onion, broccoli, garlic, and ginger paste, and cook and stir for 3 minutes.

Stir in hoisin sauce and toss well. Add salmon, and flake it with a fork into chunks. Toss; remove from heat. Add carrots and serve over rice.

Salmon Couscous Salad

Ingredients

Dressing:

1/2 cup mayonnaise

1/2 cup buttermilk

1/4 cup prepared pesto

1 lemon, juiced

1 clove garlic

ground black pepper to taste

Couscous:

1 (5.8 ounce) package herb and garlic couscous

Salmon:

1/2 pound salmon filet, with skin

1 teaspoon Greek seasoning, such as Cavender's® Greek Seasoning

1 teaspoon butter

1 teaspoon olive oil

Salad:

2 Roma tomatoes, seeded and chopped

2 cups arugula and spinach salad mix, roughly chopped

2 tablespoons shredded Parmesan cheese

2 tablespoons pepitas

How to Make

Add mayonnaise, buttermilk, pesto, lemon juice, and garlic to the bowl of a food processor. Blend until smooth. Season to taste with black pepper. Set dressing aside.

Meanwhile, heat a skillet over medium-high heat. Season salmon with Greek seasoning. Cut salmon into two filets. Melt butter in a skillet over medium heat and add olive oil. Place salmon, skin side down, in the hot skillet. Cook until salmon flakes easily with a fork, about 8 minutes.

Bring water to a boil in a saucepan; remove from heat and stir couscous into the water. Cover saucepan and let stand until water is absorbed completely, about 10 minutes.

To assemble, place salad mixture into 2 dinner bowls, and sprinkle chopped tomatoes over the salad. Fluff couscous with a fork. Mound couscous in the center of each bowl. Sprinkle Parmesan cheese around couscous. Place a salmon filet to the side of the couscous. Pour 1 to 2 tablespoons pesto dressing on top of dish. Sprinkle with pepitas. Serve immediately.

Quick Note

Nutrition data for this recipe includes the full amount of dressing ingredients. The actual amount of dressing consumed will vary

Spicy Canned Salmon Salad Rice Bowl

Ingredients

1 cup chopped English cucumber

1 tablespoon low-sodium soy sauce

1 (14 3/4 ounce) can pink salmon, skin and bone removed, drained and flaked

2 ½ tablespoons chile-garlic sauce (such as Sriracha®)

1 tablespoon light mayonnaise

1 tablespoon rice vinegar

1 cup cooked white rice

1 avocado - peeled, pitted, and sliced

1/2 teaspoon sesame seeds

1 tablespoon chopped green onion for garnish (optional)

How to Make

Combine chopped cucumbers and soy sauce in a small bowl and set aside.

In a small bowl, combine the salmon, Sriracha®, mayonnaise, and rice vinegar.

In a bowl place cooked rice and top it with the salmon mixture, sliced avocado, and chopped cucumber mixture. Sprinkle with sesame seeds. Top with extra Sriracha and green onions if desired.

Insalata di Riso (Italian Rice Salad)

Ingredients

3 cups water

1 ½ cups long-grain rice

1 large carrot, diced

½ cup frozen peas

salt to taste

¾ cup cubed prosciutto cotto (cooked ham)

¾ cup diced Swiss cheese

½ cup button mushrooms in oil, drained

⅓ cup canned corn, drained

⅓ cup sliced green olives

⅓ cup sliced black olives

⅓ cup diced pickle

⅓ cup sliced marinated artichoke hearts, drained

1 ½ tablespoons extra-virgin olive oil

1 teaspoon thyme

1 teaspoon oregano

1 (3 ounce) can tuna, drained

4 hard-boiled eggs, quartered

How to Make

Combine water, rice, carrot, peas, and salt in a saucepan. Bring to a boil; reduce heat and simmer until rice is tender but still firm to the bite, about 14 minutes. Drain excess water; let cool, 10 to 15 minutes.

Mix prosciutto cotto, Swiss cheese, button mushrooms, corn, green olives, black olives, pickle, artichoke hearts, olive oil, thyme, and oregano together in a large bowl. Stir in cooled rice mixture. Fold tuna into the salad.

Divide salad among 4 serving plates; garnish with hard-boiled eggs. Chill before serving, at least 30 minutes.

Sorghum, Quail Egg, Avocado, Kumato®and Buffalo Mozzarella Bowl

Ingredients

3 cups water

1 cup sorghum grain

5 quail eggs

½ teaspoon Sriracha salt, or to taste

¼ teaspoon ground cumin

2 tablespoons avocado oil, divided

½ teaspoon vinegar

4 ounces fresh buffalo mozzarella

4 fresh basil leaves

1 avocado, sliced

1 Kumato® tomato, diced

4 radishes, sliced

How to Make

Bring water and sorghum to a boil in a saucepan. Reduce heat to medium-low, cover, and simmer until sorghum is tender and liquid has been absorbed, about 1 hour.

Place eggs in a saucepan and fill with water; boil for 4 minutes. Remove from heat, cover, and let sit for 5 minutes.

Mix sorghum, Sriracha salt, and cumin together in a bowl. Drizzle 1 tablespoon avocado oil and vinegar over sorghum mixture and mix well; divide between 2 bowls.

Rinse quail eggs under cold water; peel and cut each egg in half. Set egg halves on top of sorghum mixture.

Shred mozzarella cheese using your hands; divide between the 2 bowls of sorghum. Tear basil leaves and sprinkle over mozzarella cheese. Divide avocado, tomato, and radishes between the bowls.

Cheryl's Veggie-Nut Patties

Ingredients

⅔ cup 1/2-inch butternut squash cubes

½ cup chopped cauliflower

½ cup chopped broccoli

½ cup raw walnuts

¼ cup raw almonds

¼ cup raw sunflower seed kernels

½ teaspoon salt

¼ teaspoon ground cumin

⅛ teaspoon ground black pepper

1 tablespoon vegetable oil

How to Make

Place a steamer insert into a saucepan and fill with water to just below the bottom of the steamer. Bring water to a boil. Add butternut squash cubes, cover, and steam until tender, 7 to 10 minutes. Transfer squash to a bowl and mash; measure 1/2 cup mashed squash and reserve.

Place the steamer insert back into the saucepan and refill with water to reach just below the bottom of the steamer. Bring water to a boil. Add cauliflower and broccoli, cover, and steam until tender, 2 to 6 minutes.

Process walnuts, almonds, and sunflower seeds together in a blender or food processor until mixture resembles coarse breadcrumbs. Add broccoli and cauliflower, blend until finely chopped and incorporated.

Blend 1/2 cup mashed squash, salt, cumin, and black pepper into the nuts mixture until well-mixed. If mixture is too thick to process, transfer it to a bowl and mix by hand.

Divide mixture into 4 equal portions and shape into patties.

Heat oil in a large skillet over medium-high heat. Cook patties in hot oil until browned and heated through, about 2 minutes per side.

Quick Note

You can use any combination of desired nuts and seeds to equal 1 cup.

For even more flavor, toast the nuts in a dry skillet over medium heat for a few minutes until fragrant and lightly browned.

Cooked pumpkin might work as a substitute for the butternut squash.

For a shortcut, use a frozen (defrosted) cauliflower/broccoli mix.

Quinoa Pilaf with Veggies and Chickpeas

Ingredients

4 cups chicken stock

2 cups quinoa

2 tablespoons olive oil

1 pound asparagus, chopped

2 green bell peppers, chopped

1 red onion, chopped

1 (14.5 ounce) can chickpeas, drained and rinsed

2 tablespoons balsamic vinegar (Optional)

1 tablespoon lemon juice

salt and ground black pepper to taste

1 tablespoon balsamic vinegar, or more to taste (Optional)

How to Make

Combine chicken stock and quinoa in a saucepan and bring to a boil. Reduce heat to medium-low, cover, and simmer until quinoa is tender, about 15 minutes. Remove from heat.

Heat olive oil in a large skillet over medium heat until shimmering. Add asparagus, bell peppers, and onion; cook and stir until softened, about 6 minutes. Stir in chickpeas. Pour in 2 tablespoons balsamic vinegar and cook until reduced, about 4 minutes. Add lemon juice, salt, and black pepper.

Stir in cooked quinoa. Drizzle 1 tablespoon balsamic vinegar over pilaf before serving.

Quick Note

Substitute red or orange bell peppers for the green if preferred.

Tempeh Gyros

Ingredients

1 cup vegetable broth

2 tablespoons soy sauce

2 tablespoons lemon juice

2 teaspoons dried oregano

2 teaspoons ground thyme

1 ½ teaspoons minced garlic

1 (8 ounce) package tempeh

4 (6 inch) whole-wheat pitas

1 dash pink Himalayan salt

1 dash ground black pepper

Tzatziki:

2 small cucumbers, peeled and grated

1 (12.3 ounce) package silken tofu

1 tablespoon (packed) fresh dill

1 teaspoon minced fresh garlic

salt and ground black pepper to taste

2 tomatoes, sliced

½ red onion, thinly sliced

How to Make

Combine vegetable broth, soy sauce, lemon juice, oregano, thyme, 1 1/2 teaspoons garlic, Himalayan salt, and dash of pepper in a large bowl.

Bring a saucepan of water to a boil. Cut tempeh in half and add to the boiling water. Boil for 10 minutes to remove any bitter taste. Transfer tempeh to a cutting board and allow to cool slightly.

Cut tempeh into 1/4-inch slices and place them in the vegetable broth marinade. Cover with plastic wrap and marinate in the refrigerator 8 hours to overnight, stirring occasionally to be sure tempeh is covered with marinade.

Preheat oven to 400 degrees F (200 degrees C). Line a baking sheet with parchment paper.

Transfer marinated tempeh slices to the prepared baking sheet.

Bake in the preheated oven, turning halfway through, until golden brown and beginning to crisp at the edges, 30 to 35 minutes.

Place pitas in the hot oven until warmed through, 3 to 5 minutes.

Squeeze excess water from cucumbers using a paper towel. Place tofu, cucumbers, dill, 1 teaspoon garlic, salt, and pepper in a food processor. Blend until tzatziki is well mixed. Adjust seasonings if desired.

Assemble a gyro by placing 1/4 of tempeh slices, tomatoes, and red onions on top of a pita. Cover with tzatziki. Repeat with remaining tempeh, tomatoes, onion, and pita.

Quick Note

Use tamari instead of soy sauce and gluten-free pita in place of whole wheat pita for a gluten-free version.

Whole wheat pita can also be substituted with sprouted wheat pita.

For non-vegan version of tzatziki, use about 1 cup plain Greek yogurt in place of the tofu.

Spicy Chicken Noodle Soup

Ingredients

2 skinless, boneless chicken breast halves, diced

2 cloves garlic, minced

6 cups vegetable broth

3 carrots, sliced

½ cup frozen corn

1 (8 ounce) package dried thin rice noodles

1 red bell pepper, diced

1 teaspoon dried basil

½ teaspoon chili pepper flakes, or to taste

How to Make

Cook and stir chicken in a large pot over medium heat until lightly browned, about 5 minutes; stir in garlic and cook until fragrant, about 1 minute.

Stir vegetable broth, carrots, and corn into chicken mixture; bring to a boil. Stir rice noodles, red pepper, basil, and chili flakes into chicken mixture;

reduce heat and simmer until noodles are tender, about 5 minutes.

Quick Note

This recipe can easily be modified to be gluten-free by using the appropriate gluten-free soup base. Also feel free to throw in any vegetables that you enjoy- it always tastes fantastic!

Chicken and Veggie Quinoa Bowls

Ingredients

2 cups chicken broth

1 cup quinoa

salt and ground black pepper to taste

2 tablespoons olive oil

1 green bell pepper, chopped

½ yellow onion, chopped

2 zucchinis, chopped

1 clove garlic, minced

1 head broccoli, chopped

1 pint grape tomatoes, halved

1 pound rotisserie chicken, boned and chopped

1 (5.5 ounce) package crumbled goat cheese

1 avocado, sliced

1 lemon, juiced

How to Make

Bring chicken broth and quinoa to a boil in a saucepan. Reduce heat to medium-low, cover, and simmer until quinoa is tender, 15 to 20 minutes. Season with salt and pepper.

While quinoa cooks, heat olive oil in a pan over low heat until gleaming. Add bell pepper and onion and saute for 1 to 2 minutes. Turn heat to medium-high, add zucchinis and garlic, and saute until they are starting to soften and the onion is transparent, 5 to 7 minutes. Add broccoli and saute until bright green. Season veggies with salt and pepper. Stir in tomatoes and quickly saute until they start to crinkle and soften, about 5 minutes. Add chicken to warm through, about 5 minutes more.

Separate the quinoa into 6 bowls and top with desired amount of veggies. Top with goat cheese, avocado, and lemon juice.

Quick Note

You can use any kind of cooked, shredded chicken you prefer. You can use vegetable broth instead of chicken.

The avocado, goat cheese, and lemon juice are optional for topping.

DINNER RECIPES FOR CSID

Grilled Marinated Swordfish

Ingredients

Marinade:

⅓ cup white wine

¼ cup lemon juice

2 tablespoons soy sauce

2 tablespoons olive oil

4 cloves garlic

1 tablespoon poultry seasoning

¼ teaspoon salt

⅛ teaspoon pepper

Other:

4 swordfish steaks

1 tablespoon chopped fresh parsley (Optional)

4 slices lemon, for garnish (Optional)

How to Make

To make the marinade: Mix wine, lemon juice, soy sauce, olive oil, garlic, poultry seasoning, salt, and pepper in a glass baking dish until combined.

Lay swordfish steaks in marinade; turn to coat. Refrigerate for 1 hour, turning frequently.

Preheat an outdoor grill for high heat and lightly oil the grate.

Cook swordfish steaks on the preheated grill until cooked through and the fish flakes easily with a fork, 5 to 6 minutes per side; discard marinade. An instant-read thermometer inserted into the center of each steak should read at least 145 degrees F (63 degrees C).

Garnish swordfish steaks with parsley and serve with lemon wedges.

Persian Fried Fish with Saffron and Turmeric

Ingredients

1/4 teaspoon ground saffron

3 tablespoons lemon juice (from 1 lemon)

2 tablespoons olive oil

2 teaspoons salt, divided

1 teaspoon black pepper, divided

8 (6-oz.) white fish fillets, such as mahi-mahi, haddock, or flounder

1 cup flour

1 teaspoon turmeric

1 teaspoon paprika

1/4 cup vegetable oil

lemon wedges, for serving

How to Make

To bloom saffron, sprinkle saffron over a few ice cubes in a small bowl; let stand at room temperature until ice melts completely, about 45 minutes.

For marinade, stir together saffron mixture, lemon juice, olive oil, 1 teaspoon salt, and 1/2 teaspoon pepper in a small bowl. Put fish in a shallow dish; pour marinade over fish, turning to coat. Cover and marinate in the refrigerator for 20 minutes. (Avoid marinating longer, which can cause the fish to "cook" in the acidic mixture.)

Stir together flour, turmeric, paprika, and remaining 1 teaspoon salt and 1/2 teaspoon pepper in a shallow dish.

Heat vegetable oil in a very large skillet over medium heat.

Dredge fish in flour mixture, coating both sides of each fillet. Working in batches as needed, fry fish in the hot oil, turning once, until fish flakes easily with a fork, 5 to 7 minutes. An instant-read thermometer inserted into the center should read at least 145 degrees F (63 degrees C).

Transfer fish to a wire rack. Serve immediately with lemon wedges.

Note

Sabzi Khordan:

A platter of feta, nuts, veggies, and piles of fresh herbs is a quintessential accessory to most Persian meals—it plays the part of salad, appetizer, and serve-yourself dinner garnishes, all at once.

Quick Air Fryer Tilapia

Ingredients

olive oil cooking spray

2 tablespoons all-purpose flour

1 ½ teaspoons seafood seasoning (such as Old Bay®)

¾ teaspoon paprika

½ teaspoon garlic powder

salt and freshly ground black pepper to taste

1 pound tilapia fillets, thawed if frozen

4 lemon slices

How to Make

Preheat an air fryer to 400 degrees F (200 degrees C). Spray the air fryer basket with olive oil spray or line with a parchment liner.

Whisk flour, seafood seasoning, paprika, garlic powder, salt, and pepper together in a small bowl.

Remove tilapia filets from the package and pat dry with a paper towel. Lightly spray filets with olive oil, and sprinkle flour seasoning over each filet, pressing down to coat all of the fish. Turn them over, and season on the other side as well. Place the filets into the air fryer basket, without overlapping, so air can circulate around the filets.

Cook until tilapia filets flake easily with a fork, 7 to 10 minutes. There is no need to flip them. Depending on your air fryer size, you might have to cook them in batches.

Top each filet with a slice of lemon, and serve hot.

Quick Note

Cook time may vary depending on the brand and size of your air fryer

Air Fryer Tilapia

Ingredients

½ cup freshly grated Parmesan cheese

1 ½ teaspoons paprika

1 teaspoon garlic powder

½ teaspoon salt

½ teaspoon freshly ground black pepper

4 (6 ounce) tilapia fillets, thawed if frozen

cooking spray

1 tablespoon minced fresh parsley (Optional)

4 lemon wedges (optional)

How to Make

Preheat the air fryer to 400 degrees F (200 degrees C).

Combine Parmesan cheese, paprika, garlic powder, salt, and pepper in a bowl.

Pat tilapia filets dry with paper towels. Spritz both sides with cooking spray, then press both sides of the filets into the Parmesan mixture. Shake off any excess, then spray again with cooking spray. Place in the basket of the air fryer.

Cook until the fish flakes easily with a fork, 6 to 8 minutes. You may need to cook the fish in 2 batches, depending on the size of your air fryer.

Sprinkle with parsley and serve with lemon wedges.

Quick Note

This recipe was developed using a 5 quart basket-style air fryer. Cooking time may vary if using a different style or size.

Maple Mustard Salmon

Ingredients

2 ½ tablespoons stone-ground mustard

1 tablespoon maple syrup

1 teaspoon fresh lemon juice

½ teaspoon minced garlic

¼ teaspoon minced fresh thyme

6 (6 ounce) frozen salmon fillets, thawed and patted dry

1 teaspoon kosher salt

½ teaspoon black pepper

1 tablespoon olive oil

How to Make

Preheat the oven to 400 degrees F (200 degrees C). Line a large baking sheet with foil.

Whisk together mustard, maple syrup, lemon juice, garlic, and thyme in a small bowl.

Season salmon on both sides with salt and pepper and brush with oil. Arrange salmon on prepared baking sheet. Brush with mustard mixture.

Bake in the preheated oven until salmon flakes easily with a fork, 8 to 10 minutes.

Quick Note

If your salmon has skin, arrange skin sides down on the baking sheet.

Marinated Tuna Steak

Ingredients

¼ cup orange juice

¼ cup soy sauce

2 tablespoons olive oil

2 tablespoons chopped fresh parsley

1 tablespoon lemon juice

1 clove garlic, minced

½ teaspoon chopped fresh oregano

½ teaspoon ground black pepper

4 (4 ounce) tuna steaks

How to Make

Mix orange juice, soy sauce, olive oil, parsley, lemon juice, garlic, oregano, and pepper together in a large non-reactive dish until well combined. Place tuna steaks in marinade and turn to coat.

Cover the dish with plastic wrap and marinate in the refrigerator for at least 30 minutes.

Preheat an outdoor grill for high heat and lightly oil the grate. Remove tuna steaks from the marinade and shake off excess; reserve marinade for basting.

Cook tuna steaks on the preheated grill for 5 to 6 minutes; flip steaks and baste with reserved marinade. Cook for an additional 5 minutes, or to desired doneness. Discard any remaining marinade.

Vegan Jamaican Curry

Ingredients

2 tablespoons grapeseed oil

1 (14 ounce) package tofu, cut into bite-sized cubes

1 yellow onion, chopped

1 red bell pepper, chopped

2 to 3 tablespoons Jamaican yellow curry powder, divided

1 small zucchini, cut into bite-sized pieces

1/2 cup sliced cremini mushrooms or baby bellas

1/4 cup coconut milk

salt and freshly ground black pepper to taste

How to Make

Heat grapeseed oil in a cast iron skillet over medium-high heat. Pat excess water from tofu with a paper towel, and fry tofu in the hot skillet until browned around the edges, about 4 minutes per side. Remove from skillet and set aside.

Add onions, bell peppers, and 1 tablespoon curry powder to the skillet and sauté for 2 minutes. Add zucchini and mushrooms to the skillet; sauté for 3 minutes.

Return tofu to the skillet, add 1 tablespoon curry powder, or more to taste, and mix well. Pour in coconut milk, stir well. Reduce heat to low, cover, and let simmer for 3 to 5 minutes. Season with salt and pepper.

Lemon, Ricotta, and Spinach Pasta

Ingredients

1 pound fusilli corti bucati pasta

1 cup ricotta cheese

1/2 cup olive oil

1/2 cup freshly grated Parmesan cheese, plus more for serving

2 lemons, zested and juiced

1 teaspoon salt, or to taste

1 teaspoon Italian seasoning

1/2 teaspoon garlic powder

1/2 teaspoon freshly ground black pepper

1 pinch crushed red pepper flakes

2 cups baby spinach

small handful basil leaves, cut into very thin strips, or to taste

1 teaspoon fresh thyme, or to taste

lemon slices

How to Make

Bring a large pot of lightly salted water to a boil. Add fusilli and return to a boil; cook until pasta is tender with a bite, 8 to 12 minutes. Reserve 2 cups pasta water, then drain. Return pasta to the pot.

In a medium bowl, stir together ricotta, olive oil, Parmesan cheese, lemon juice, and lemon zest. Season with Italian seasoning, garlic granules, salt, black pepper, and a pinch of red pepper flakes.

Add ricotta mixture and 1/4 cup reserved pasta water to pasta and toss. The sauce will thicken and adhere as it is tossed. Add more reserved pasta water if the sauce is too thick.

Place spinach in a colander. Pour remaining reserved pasta water over spinach to wilt; toss spinach into pasta.

Divide into serving bowls. Top each serving with a slice of lemon, basil, thyme, cheese and a drizzle of olive oil, if desired

Pasta alla Trapanese (Sicilian Tomato Pesto)

Ingredients

1/2 cup whole roasted almonds

4 cloves garlic

1 teaspoon kosher salt, plus more to taste

1 cup grated pecorino Romano cheese, plus more to taste

1 cup packed fresh basil leaves

4 mint leaves (optional)

1/2 cup extra virgin olive oil

1 pound red cherry tomatoes or red grape tomatoes

1 pound busiate pasta, or other curly shaped pasta, such as fusilli

How to Make

Bring about 2 cups of water to a boil, remove from the heat, and stir in almonds; let sit for 3 to 4 minutes. Drain, and once cool enough to handle, rub skins off with your hands; alternately; transfer drained almonds to a kitchen towel, then fold up the towel and rub almonds until skins come off.

Crush sliced garlic with kosher salt in a mortar and pestle into a smooth paste. Alternately, place garlic on a board and sprinkle kosher salt on top; use the flat side of the knife to flatten, mash, and scrape the garlic and salt mixture until it is a smooth paste.

Add peeled almonds to the jar of a blender, followed by the cheese, basil, mint, garlic paste, oil, and tomatoes. Add the **Ingredients** in this order, so that the almonds and cheese have a chance to grind before the wetter **Ingredients** mix in.

Begin to pulse blender on and off until almonds and cheese are ground, then continue to pulse until remaining **Ingredients** are incorporated. Blend on high until the pesto is as coarse or smooth as you like.

Taste for salt, and adjust. Set aside while pasta is cooking.

Bring a large pot of lightly salted water to a boil. Cook busiate pasta in the boiling water, stirring occasionally, until tender yet firm to the bite, about 12 minutes. Transfer pasta into a bowl with a strainer. Reserve starchy cooking liquid.

Add about 1/3 cup of the pasta water into the bowl, and then transfer in the pesto, along with a large pinch of salt, and toss to coat. More pasta water can be added to adjust the texture. Once mixed, add another optional handful of cheese, and toss one last time. Serve immediately.

Farro Salad with Pecans, Feta, and Cherries

Ingredients

2 cups water

1 cup farro

½ cup chopped celery

⅓ cup crumbled feta cheese

¼ cup dried cherries

¼ cup chopped green onions

2 tablespoons chopped toasted pecans

½ teaspoon lemon zest

1 ½ tablespoons lemon juice

1 tablespoon extra-virgin olive oil

¼ teaspoon salt

¼ teaspoon freshly ground black pepper

lemon wedges for serving

How to Make

Combine water, farro, and salt in a small saucepan and bring to a boil. Cover and simmer over low heat until water is absorbed, about 20 minutes.

Drain, spread on a baking sheet, and chill 5 minutes.

Mix celery, feta, dried cherries, green onion, pecans, lemon zest, lemon juice, olive oil, salt, and pepper in a bowl. Add farro; toss to combine. Serve with lemon wedges.

Black Beans and Rice

Ingredients

1 teaspoon olive oil

1 onion, chopped

2 cloves garlic, minced

¾ cup uncooked white rice

1 ½ cups low sodium, low fat vegetable broth

3 ½ cups canned black beans, drained

1 teaspoon ground cumin

¼ teaspoon cayenne pepper

How to Make

Heat oil in a saucepan over medium-high heat. Add onion and garlic; cook and stir until onion has softened, about 4 minutes. Stir in rice to coat; cook and stir for 2 minutes.

Add vegetable broth and bring to a boil. Cover, reduce to a simmer, and cook until liquid is absorbed, about 20 minutes.

Stir in beans, cumin, and cayenne; cook until beans are warmed through.

Mushroom Stir-Fry

Ingredients

Sauce:

3 tablespoons low-sodium soy sauce

2 tablespoons rice wine vinegar

1 tablespoon sesame oil

2 teaspoons honey

2 teaspoons cornstarch

1 teaspoon Sriracha sauce

Stir-Fry:

2 tablespoons peanut oil

2 stalks celery, thinly sliced diagonally

1 medium onion, cut into 1/2-inch wedges

¾ pound shiitake mushrooms, trimmed and cut into 1/4-inch slices

¼ pound beech mushrooms, trimmed

6 green onions, cut into 2-inch pieces, whites and greens separated and divided

¼ pound enoki mushrooms, trimmed

2 cloves garlic, minced

1 teaspoon freshly grated ginger

How to Make

Make the sauce: Whisk soy sauce, vinegar, sesame oil, honey, cornstarch, and Sriracha together in a small bowl.

Make the stir-fry: Heat peanut oil in a large wok over high heat. Add celery and onion; cook, stirring constantly, for 3 to 4 minutes. Add shiitake and beech mushrooms, and white parts from green onions; cook, stirring constantly, for 3 to 4 minutes.

Add enoki mushrooms, green parts from green onions, garlic, and ginger; stir-fry for 2 minutes. Move vegetables to one side of the wok.

Whisk sauce **Ingredients** to recombine, then pour into the empty section of the wok. Stir vegetables into the sauce and cook until thickened slightly, about 1 minute. Remove from the heat and serve immediately.

Authentic Mexican Chile Rellenos

Ingredients

6 fresh Anaheim chile peppers

1 (8 ounce) package queso asadero (white Mexican cheese), cut into 3/4-inch thick strips

2 large eggs, separated

1 teaspoon baking powder

¾ cup all-purpose flour

1 cup vegetable shortening for frying

How to Make

Preheat the oven broiler; set the oven rack about 6 inches below the heat source. Line a baking sheet with aluminum foil.

Place peppers onto the prepared baking sheet and broil until skins are blackened and blistered, about 10 minutes. Use tongs to rotate peppers often to char all sides. Place blackened peppers into a bowl and tightly seal with plastic wrap. Allow peppers to steam as they cool, about 15 minutes.

Remove skin from peppers, then cut a slit down the long side of each one to remove seeds and core. Rinse peppers inside and out and pat dry with paper towels. Stuff peppers with strips of cheese.

Whisk egg yolks and baking powder in a bowl until combined. Beat egg whites with an electric mixer in a separate bowl until stiff peaks form. Gently fold beaten whites into the yolk mixture. Place flour into a separate shallow bowl.

Melt vegetable shortening in a skillet over medium heat. Roll each stuffed pepper in flour, tap off excess flour, and dip into the egg mixture to coat both sides. Gently lay coated peppers into the hot shortening. Fry peppers until lightly golden brown and cheese has melted, about 5 minutes per side.

MAIN DISHES RECIPES FOR CSID

Baked Asian Rockfish

Ingredients

4 (6 ounce) rockfish filets

1 tablespoon sesame oil

2 cloves garlic, minced

1 tablespoon finely minced fresh ginger

1 tablespoon honey

1/4 teaspoon red pepper flakes

1 tablespoon soy sauce

1 tablespoon lime juice

1/4 cup diagonally thinly sliced scallions

How to Make

Preheat the oven to 400 degrees F (200 degrees C).
Line a shallow baking pan with aluminum foil, and

spray with cooking spray. Place filets onto the prepared baking pan.

In a small bowl combine sesame oil, soy sauce, lime juice, honey, ginger, garlic, and pepper flakes. Spoon mixture evenly over top of filets.

Bake in the preheated oven until fish flakes easily with a fork, 10 to 15 minutes. Sprinkle filets with scallions before serving.

Baked Whole Crappie

Ingredients

4 whole crappie fish, gutted and cleaned, tails still on

1 bunch fresh cilantro

1/4 cup extra virgin olive oil

2 tablespoons lime juice

3 cloves garlic

2 teaspoons salt

1 teaspoon paprika

8 thin lemon slices

How to Make

Preheat the oven to 400 degrees F (200 degrees C). Line a shallow baking pan with aluminum foil.

Pat fish dry; score the skin of fish in a diamond pattern with a very sharp knife. Place fish on the prepared baking pan. Cover tails of fish with aluminum foil to avoid overbrowning.

Combine cilantro, olive oil, lime juice, garlic, salt, and paprika in a blender; pulse until mixture is a soft paste.

Spread cilantro-garlic paste on each fish, pressing the paste into the scored sections. Place 2 lemon slices on each fish.

Bake, uncovered, in the preheated oven until fish flakes easily when tested with a fork, about 20 minutes.

Easy Tuna Patties

Ingredients

2 eggs

2 teaspoons lemon juice

10 tablespoons Italian-seasoned bread crumbs

3 tablespoons grated Parmesan cheese

3 (5 ounce) cans tuna, drained

3 tablespoons diced onion

1 pinch ground black pepper

3 tablespoons vegetable oil

How to Make

Beat eggs and lemon juice in a bowl; stir in bread crumbs and Parmesan cheese to make a paste. Fold in tuna and onion until well combined; season with black pepper.

Use your hands to shape tuna mixture into 8 (1-inch-thick) patties.

Heat vegetable oil in a skillet over medium heat. Fry patties in the hot oil until golden brown, about 5 minutes per side.

Simple Broiled Haddock

Ingredients

2 pounds haddock fillets

½ teaspoon onion powder

½ teaspoon paprika

½ teaspoon garlic powder

½ teaspoon ground black pepper

½ teaspoon salt

¼ teaspoon cayenne pepper

1 tablespoon butter, cut in small pieces

1 lemon, cut into wedges

How to Make

Set an oven rack about 6 inches from the heat source and preheat the oven's broiler. Line a baking sheet with aluminum foil; spray with cooking spray.

Arrange haddock fillets on the prepared baking sheet.

Mix onion powder, paprika, garlic powder, black pepper, salt, and cayenne pepper in a small bowl; sprinkle seasoning over fish, then dot with butter.

Broil in the preheated oven until fish flakes easily with a fork, 6 to 8 minutes. Serve with lemon wedges.

Fish in Foil

Ingredients

2 rainbow trout fillets

1 tablespoon olive oil

2 teaspoons garlic salt

1 teaspoon ground black pepper

2 sheets heavy-duty aluminum foil

1 fresh jalapeno pepper, sliced

1 lemon, sliced

How to Make

Preheat the oven to 400 degrees F (200 degrees C).

Rinse and pat fillets dry. Rub fillets with olive oil, and season with garlic salt and black pepper. Place each fillet on a large sheet of aluminum foil. Top with jalapeno slices, and squeeze the juice from the ends of the lemon over fillets. Arrange remaining lemon slices on top of fillets.

Carefully seal all edges of the foil to form enclosed packets. Place packets on a baking sheet.

Bake in the preheated oven until fish flakes easily with a fork, 15 to 20 minutes depending on size of fillets.

Grilled Cod

Ingredients

2 (8 ounce) fillets cod, cut in half

1 tablespoon Cajun seasoning

½ teaspoon lemon pepper

¼ teaspoon salt

¼ teaspoon ground black pepper

2 tablespoons butter

1 lemon, juiced

2 tablespoons chopped green onion (white part only)

How to Make

Stack about 15 charcoal briquettes into a grill in a pyramid shape. If desired, drizzle coals lightly with lighter fluid and allow to soak for 1 minute before lighting coals with a match. Allow fire to spread to all coals, about 10 minutes, before spreading briquettes out into the grill; let coals burn until a thin layer of white ash covers the coals. Lightly oil the grates.

Season both sides of cod fillets with Cajun seasoning, lemon pepper, salt, and black pepper. Set fillets aside on a plate.

Melt butter in a small saucepan over medium heat, stir in lemon juice and green onion, and cook until onion is softened, about 3 minutes.

Grill fillets on the preheated grill until browned and flaky, about 3 minutes per side; baste frequently with butter mixture while grilling.

Allow fillets to rest off the heat for about 5 minutes before serving.

Cabbage Fried Rice

Ingredients

3 large eggs

1/8 teaspoon salt

1/4 teaspoon freshly ground black pepper

2 1/2 tablespoons sesame oil, divided

3 cloves garlic, minced

1 small yellow onion, chopped

1 small green pepper, chopped

3 cups shredded cabbage

2 cups leftover cooked white rice

3 tablespoons soy sauce

2 teaspoons grated fresh ginger

1 pinch red pepper flakes (optional)

1 green onion, thinly sliced (optional)

How to Make

In a bowl, whisk eggs with salt and pepper.

Heat a large skillet over medium high heat; add 1/2 tablespoon sesame oil. Cook and stir eggs in the hot oil until scrambled and set, 3 to 4 minutes. Transfer eggs to a plate, clean the pan, and return to medium high heat.

Pour in remaining 2 tablespoons sesame oil, then add garlic and cook for 1 minute. Stir in onions and green peppers and cook for about 5 minutes. Add cabbage and cook until softened, about 5 minutes more.

Stir in cooked rice, soy sauce, grated ginger, and cooked eggs. Stir until combined and heated thoroughly, about 5 minutes. Add red pepper flakes and top with green onions. Serve warm.

Creamy Wild Mushroom Risotto

Ingredients

2 ounces dried chanterelle mushrooms

1 ½ teaspoons butter

1 teaspoon truffle oil (Optional)

1 chopped onion

2 shallots, minced

1 clove garlic, minced

3 ounces sliced fresh button mushrooms

1 (12 ounce) package Arborio rice

½ cup dry white wine

1 quart hot chicken stock

2 tablespoons heavy cream

2 tablespoons crumbled Gorgonzola cheese, or to taste

ground black pepper to taste

How to Make

Cover chanterelle mushrooms with hot water, cover, and set aside to soften for 30 minutes. Once soft, remove mushrooms from water and chop; discard water.

Melt butter along with truffle oil in a large saucepan over medium-high heat. Add onion, shallot, and garlic; cook and stir two minutes until the onion begins to soften. Add fresh mushrooms; continue cooking until mushroom softens and begin to release their liquid. Stir in chopped chanterelle mushrooms, and cook 3 minutes more.

Add Arborio rice; cook and stir for a few minutes until rice looks glossy and is well coated with onion mixture. Stir in white wine and cook until nearly evaporated.

Reduce heat to medium; add 1/3 of the hot chicken stock. Cook and stir until chicken stock has been mostly absorbed, about 5 minutes. The risotto should be simmering gently while you stir in chicken stock. Add 1/2 of the remaining stock, and stir for 5 minutes more. Finally add remaining stock, and continue cooking until risotto is creamy and rice is tender, about 5 minutes more. The rice should not be completely soft, but still have a little firmness when you bite into it. You can add a little water if needed to cook the rice to this state.

Remove risotto from the heat, and stir in heavy cream and Gorgonzola cheese. Season to taste with salt and pepper, and serve.

Easy Kimchi Fried Rice

Ingredients

1 tablespoon butter

1 tablespoon olive oil

3 drops sesame oil, or to taste

¼ cup diced onion

¼ cup shredded carrots

2 scallions, white and light green parts, sliced

½ cup cubed, fully cooked ham

⅓ cup chopped kimchi

1 teaspoon garlic powder

2 cups cooked rice

1 tablespoon soy sauce

1 tablespoon gochujang (Korean chile paste)

salt and ground black pepper to taste

How to Make

Warm butter and olive oil together over medium-high heat in a large skillet or wok. Add in sesame oil. Add onion, carrots, and scallions and cook until onion is translucent, about 2 minutes. Mix in cubed ham and kimchi; cook for 1 more minute. Season with garlic powder.

Stir in rice and cook until mixture is heated throughout. Drizzle soy sauce over top and mix in gochujang. Stir until well combined and adjust seasoning with salt and pepper.

Garlic Chicken, Vegetable and Rice Skillet

Ingredients

1 serving Vegetable cooking spray

1 ¼ pounds skinless, boneless chicken breast halves

2 cloves garlic, minced

1 ¾ cups Swanson® Chicken Broth or Swanson® Chicken Stock

¾ cup uncooked white rice

1 (16 ounce) package frozen vegetable combination (broccoli, cauliflower, carrots)

⅓ cup grated Parmesan cheese

1 teaspoon Paprika

How to Make

Spray a 12-inch skillet with the cooking spray and heat over medium-high heat for 1 minute. Add the chicken and garlic and cook for 10 minutes or until the chicken is well browned on both sides. Remove the chicken from the skillet.

Stir the broth, rice and vegetables in the skillet and heat to a boil. Reduce the heat to low. Cover and cook for 15 minutes. Stir in the cheese.

Return the chicken to the skillet. Sprinkle the chicken with the paprika. Cover and cook for 10 minutes or until the chicken is cooked through and the rice is tender.

Air Fryer Shrimp Fried Rice

Ingredients

1 tablespoon canola oil

1/3 cup chopped onion

1/3 cup chopped carrot

1 teaspoon kosher salt, divided

2 large eggs, lightly beaten

1 pound large, peeled, deveined raw shrimp

2 (8-ounce) packages pre-cooked microwavable brown rice

3/4 cup frozen green peas

1 tablespoon soy sauce

1 teaspoon rice vinegar

1/4 teaspoon freshly ground black pepper

1 tablespoon toasted sesame seeds, or as needed (optional)

1/4 cup Sriracha mayonnaise, or as needed

1 scallion, sliced, or as needed

How to Make

Remove the basket insert from air fryer. Preheat the air fryer to 400 degrees F (200 degrees C) for 5 minutes.

Add oil to the basket holder to coat; add onion, carrot, and 1/2 teaspoon of the salt, and stir to combine. Cook for 5 minutes. Add eggs; cook until partially set, about 3 minutes.

Add shrimp, rice, peas, soy sauce, vinegar, pepper, and remaining salt to egg mixture; stir to combine. Cook for 10 minutes. Stir mixture, sprinkle with sesame seeds, if desired, and cook until heated throughout and crisp, 10 to 15 minutes more.

Drizzle with Sriracha mayonnaise, and sprinkle with scallions.

Arroz Con Pollo (Chicken and Rice)

Ingredients

4 skinless, boneless chicken breast halves, cut into 1-inch pieces

½ teaspoon salt, divided

½ teaspoon ground black pepper, divided

½ teaspoon paprika, divided

3 tablespoons vegetable oil

1 green bell pepper, chopped

¾ cup chopped onion

1 ½ teaspoons minced garlic

1 cup long-grain white rice

1 (14.5 ounce) can chicken broth

1 (14.5 ounce) can stewed tomatoes

½ cup white wine

⅛ teaspoon saffron

1 tablespoon chopped fresh parsley

How to Make

Season chicken with a 1/4 teaspoon of salt, 1/4 teaspoon pepper, and 1/4 teaspoon paprika.

Heat oil in a large skillet over medium heat. Add seasoned chicken; cook and stir until no longer pink in the center and golden brown on all sides, about 10 minutes. Transfer chicken onto a plate; set aside.

Add green pepper, onions, and garlic to the same skillet; cook and stir for 5 minutes. Add rice; cook and stir until rice is opaque, 1 to 2 minutes. Stir in broth, tomatoes, white wine, and saffron. Stir in remaining 1/4 teaspoon salt, 1/4 teaspoon pepper, and 1/4 teaspoon paprika; bring to a boil, cover, and simmer for 20 minutes.

Add chicken and stir until heated through. Stir in parsley and serve.

Buffalo Chicken Dynamite Rice

Ingredients

6 boneless, skinless chicken thighs

2 tablespoons melted butter

salt to taste

⅔ cup mayonnaise

3 tablespoons hot pepper sauce (such as Frank's RedHot®)

1 teaspoon cayenne pepper, or more to taste

½ teaspoon paprika

¼ teaspoon garlic powder

¼ teaspoon freshly ground black pepper

1 tablespoon white vinegar

1 cup long grain rice, cooked according to package directions

1 cup diced celery, divided

½ cup crumbled blue cheese, divided

How to Make

Preheat the oven to 400 degrees F (200 degrees C).

Add chicken thighs and melted butter to a baking dish, and toss until coated. Season the top with salt.

Bake in the preheated oven until chicken is just cooked through, about 20 minutes.

While chicken is cooking, make sauce by adding mayonnaise, hot sauce, cayenne pepper, paprika, garlic powder, black pepper and white vinegar to a mixing bowl. Whisk together, and refrigerate until ready to use.

Remove cooked chicken from the oven. Transfer thighs to a plate or bowl, and place in the fridge until needed. Reserve all the juices and drippings from the casserole dish, and pour into a measuring cup. Add enough water to get to 1 2/3 cups.

Bring water-drippings mixture and rice to a boil in a saucepan. Reduce heat to medium-low, cover, and simmer until rice is tender and water has been absorbed, about 15 minutes. Turn off heat and allow rice to sit for 10 minutes longer.

Transfer cooked rice to the baking dish used to bake the chicken. Use a spoon to create an even layer, but do not pack or press rice down. Drizzle any accumulated sauce from the cooked chicken over the rice.

Transfer chicken to a cutting board and cut into 1/2-inch cubes. Add chicken to the mayo sauce and mix well. Sprinkle 1/2 of the celery over the rice. Spread out chicken-mayo mixture evenly over the rice. Crumble over about 1/2 of the blue cheese and season with some cayenne on top, if desired.

Preheat the oven to 450 degrees F (230 degrees C).

Place baking dish in the preheated oven and cook until the top starts to brown, 15 to 20 minutes. For additional browning, set broiler to high, and broil top for 1 to 2 minutes to achieve more color. Garnish top with the rest of the celery, more blue cheese if desired, and another drizzle of hot sauce. Top with celery leaves if available. Serve hot, or at room temp.

Southeast Asian Style Chicken Rice

Ingredients

Chicken Rice:

1 large chicken breast, skin on

1 teaspoon kosher salt, plus more as needed

1 tablespoon vegetable oil

1 tablespoon minced ginger

2 cloves garlic, minced

⅓ cup diced onions

½ teaspoon turmeric

1 cup plus 1 tablespoon jasmine rice

1 ½ cups chicken broth

Chicken Herb Salad:

½ cup thinly sliced red onion

¼ cup sliced green onions

1 small red Fresno chili, thinly sliced, or any other hot pepper

2 tablespoons fresh lime juice, plus more to taste

2 teaspoons soy sauce, or to taste

1 teaspoon sambal hot chili sauce

1 teaspoon sesame oil, or to taste

¼ teaspoon freshly ground black pepper

salt to taste

½ cup freshly torn mint leaves

½ cup freshly torn cilantro leaves

lime wedges (Optional)

How to Make

Set chicken breast onto a cutting board and make 5 or 6 shallow cuts through the skin. Season generously on both sides with salt.

Heat vegetable oil in a skillet over medium high heat and sear chicken breast, skin-side down, until the skin is golden brown and fat has rendered out, about 5 minutes. Flip breast over, and keep cooking until chicken is cooked through, about 5 minutes more. If oil starts to smoke before the chicken is cooked, reduce heat to medium or medium-low.

Turn off the heat and transfer chicken to a plate to rest until cool enough to handle. Peel off the skin and finely chop. Refrigerate chicken breast.

Add minced chicken skin back into the skillet over and medium heat. Cook and stir until the skin browns and starts getting crisp, 3 to 5 minutes. Add ginger, garlic, and onions and cook, stirring, until onions start to turn translucent, about 5 minutes. Add turmeric and rice; cook and stir until rice is well coated with oil, 2 to 3 minutes.

Stir in broth, turn heat to high, and bring to a boil. Cover, reduce heat to low, and simmer undisturbed for 20 minutes. Turn off the heat and set a timer for 10 minutes to allow rice to rest.

Meanwhile, shred the chicken meat using your hands or cut into small pieces. Place into a bowl. Add red onion, green onions, Fresno chili, lime juice, soy sauce, hot sauce, sesame oil, salt, pepper, fresh mint and cilantro. Toss until well combined.

Taste and adjust with more lime juice, salt, and/or spice as needed.

After the 10 minute rice timer is up, remove cover, and fluff rice with a fork. Taste and adjust seasoning if necessary. Serve rice topped with the chicken herb salad mixture and lime wedges.

Easy Korean Ground Beef Bowl

Ingredients

1 pound lean ground beef

5 cloves garlic, crushed

1 tablespoon freshly grated ginger

2 teaspoons toasted sesame oil

½ cup reduced-sodium soy sauce

⅓ cup light brown sugar

¼ teaspoon crushed red pepper

6 green onions, chopped, divided

4 cups hot cooked brown rice

1 tablespoon toasted sesame seeds

How to Make

Heat a large skillet over medium-high heat. Add beef and cook, stirring and crumbling into small pieces until browned, 5 to 7 minutes. Drain excess grease.

Stir in garlic, ginger, and sesame oil and cook until fragrant, about 2 minutes. Stir in soy sauce, brown sugar, and red pepper. Cook until beef absorbs some sauce, about 7 minutes. Add 1/2 of chopped green onions.

Serve over hot cooked rice; garnish with sesame seeds and remaining green onions.

Spicy Tuna Rice Bowl

Ingredients

1 cup uncooked long-grain rice

1 ½ cups water

1 (7 ounce) jar tuna packed in olive oil

½ cup finely diced red bell pepper

¼ cup finely diced jalapeno pepper

¼ cup finely sliced green onions

⅓ cup seasoned rice vinegar

½ lemon, juiced, or to taste

2 tablespoons soy sauce

2 teaspoons Sriracha hot sauce

½ teaspoon sesame oil

1 pinch Korean red pepper flakes (gochugaru), or to taste

1 teaspoon finely sliced green onion, or to taste

How to Make

Pour rice into a heavy pot and add water; swirl to allow rice to settle. Bring to a simmer over medium-high heat; do not stir. Reduce heat to low, cover, and continue to simmer for 15 minutes.

While rice is cooking, place tuna into a large mixing bowl and break up with your hands or a fork. Toss in red bell pepper, jalapeno, 1/4 cup green onions, rice vinegar, lemon juice, soy sauce, Sriracha, and sesame oil. Mix with a fork until thoroughly combined.

Turn off heat and let rice sit, covered, for 10 minutes.

Fluff rice with a fork to separate the grains and break up any large clumps; transfer into the mixing bowl. Mix thoroughly with a spoon until all the **Ingredients** are evenly incorporated. Taste and adjust seasoning if needed. Serve warm, at room temperature, or cold like a rice salad, topped with red pepper flakes and 1 teaspoon green onion.

CHAPTER VII: WHY YOU MADE THE RIGHT DECISION

The genetic basis of Congenital Sucrase-Isomaltase Deficiency (CSID), making lifestyle alterations, and engaging with a healthcare team are all aspects of the difficult path that individuals undertake when managing the illness. A lack of the sugar-digesting enzymes sucrase and isomaltase characterizes CSID, an autosomal recessive disorder. Given that CSID runs in families, genetic counseling can help with planning a family and understanding how the faulty gene could be passed along.

Among the many aspects of living with CSID, dietary management stands out. Nutritionists can help you find the sweet spot between eating enough to stay healthy and avoiding the sweets that make your symptoms worse. Managing CSID involves making careful choices about portion management, meal timing, and nutrition to promote digestive comfort and satisfy nutritional needs. One treatment strategy that can help certain people even more is enzyme replacement therapy.

Beyond the plate, lifestyle advice cover mindful eating, exercise regularly, stress management, and creating a support system. By promoting both physical and emotional resilience, these suggestions add to the larger field of CSID management.

For those with CSID, seeking professional counsel becomes a compass. Experts in gastroenterology provide insight into possible treatment measures, genetic counselors help with understanding hereditary elements, and dietitians work together to create individualized meal plans. The cornerstone of proactive CSID management is maintaining open lines of contact with healthcare providers and scheduling regular checkups.

While exercise may not have an immediate effect on enzyme shortages, it does have a multiplicity of positive health effects, including those on the digestive and psychological systems. A tailored approach to holistic health is highlighted by the need of specific exercise routines that take into account the particular demands of each person with CSID.

Essential to the holistic treatment of CSID is hydration, an apparently simple yet potent component. It helps the digestive system work at its best, reduces the likelihood of certain symptoms, and improves health in general. By tailoring their hydration methods to their specific needs, people with CSID can find a way to drink enough of water without negatively impacting their digestive health.

Knowing one's genetic makeup, eating sensibly, making lifestyle changes, and seeking expert advice are all parts of the complex dance that is CSID management. In order to help persons with CSID achieve maximum health and overcome this hereditary illness, it is important to take a tailored and holistic approach.